This Planner Belongs To:

_____

Weekly Snapshot

MON:	TO DO LIST
TUE:	
WED:	
THUR:	
FRI:	
SAT:	NOTES
SUN:	

REMINDERS

My Action Plan

DATE:

TOP PRIORITIES	GOALS

ACTION STEPS   STATUS   ✓

☐
☐
☐
☐

MILESTONES & REWARDS:

THOUGHTS & REFLECTIONS::

Weekly Priority List

MON	
TUE	
WED	
THUR	
FRI	
SAT	
SUN	

Checklist

FOR: _____   DATE: _____   ✓

_____   _____ ☐

_____   _____ ☐

_____   _____ ☐

_____   _____ ☐

_____   _____ ☐

_____   _____ ☐

_____   _____ ☐

_____   _____ ☐

_____   _____ ☐

_____   _____ ☐

_____   _____ ☐

_____   _____ ☐

_____   _____ ☐

_____   _____ ☐

NOTES:

Daily Planner

DATE

TOP PRIORITIES:

APPOINTMENTS:

GOALS FOR THE DAY::

MORNING:

AFTERNOON:

EVENING:

NOTES:

Daily Planner

DATE

TOP PRIORITIES:

APPOINTMENTS:

GOALS FOR THE DAY::

MORNING:

AFTERNOON:

EVENING:

NOTES:

Daily Planner

DATE

TOP PRIORITIES:

APPOINTMENTS:

GOALS FOR THE DAY::

MORNING:

AFTERNOON:

EVENING:

NOTES:

Daily Planner

DATE

_____

TOP PRIORITIES:

MORNING:

AFTERNOON:

EVENING:

APPOINTMENTS:

NOTES:

GOALS FOR THE DAY::

Daily Planner

DATE

TOP PRIORITIES:

APPOINTMENTS:

GOALS FOR THE DAY::

MORNING:

AFTERNOON:

EVENING:

NOTES:

Daily Planner

DATE

TOP PRIORITIES:

APPOINTMENTS:

GOALS FOR THE DAY::

MORNING:

AFTERNOON:

EVENING:

NOTES:

Daily Planner

DATE

TOP PRIORITIES:

APPOINTMENTS:

GOALS FOR THE DAY::

MORNING:

AFTERNOON:

EVENING:

NOTES:

Weekly Snapshot

MON:

TUE:

WED:

THUR:

FRI:

SAT:

SUN:

TO DO LIST

NOTES

REMINDERS

My Action Plan

DATE:

TOP PRIORITIES	GOALS

ACTION STEPS   STATUS   ✓

MILESTONES & REWARDS:

THOUGHTS & REFLECTIONS::

Weekly Priority List

MON	
TUE	
WED	
THUR	
FRI	
SAT	
SUN	

Checklist

FOR: DATE: ✓

NOTES:

Daily Planner

DATE

MORNING:

TOP PRIORITIES:

AFTERNOON:

EVENING:

APPOINTMENTS:

NOTES:

GOALS FOR THE DAY::

Daily Planner

DATE

TOP PRIORITIES:

APPOINTMENTS:

GOALS FOR THE DAY::

MORNING:

AFTERNOON:

EVENING:

NOTES:

Daily Planner

DATE

TOP PRIORITIES:

APPOINTMENTS:

GOALS FOR THE DAY::

MORNING:

AFTERNOON:

EVENING:

NOTES:

Daily Planner

DATE

TOP PRIORITIES:

APPOINTMENTS:

GOALS FOR THE DAY::

MORNING:

AFTERNOON:

EVENING:

NOTES:

Daily Planner

DATE

MORNING:

TOP PRIORITIES:

AFTERNOON:

EVENING:

APPOINTMENTS:

NOTES:

GOALS FOR THE DAY::

Daily Planner

DATE

TOP PRIORITIES:

APPOINTMENTS:

GOALS FOR THE DAY::

MORNING:

AFTERNOON:

EVENING:

NOTES:

Daily Planner

DATE

MORNING:

TOP PRIORITIES:

AFTERNOON:

APPOINTMENTS:

EVENING:

NOTES:

GOALS FOR THE DAY::

Weekly Snapshot

MON:

TUE:

WED:

THUR:

FRI:

SAT:

SUN:

TO DO LIST

NOTES

REMINDERS

My Action Plan

DATE:

TOP PRIORITIES

GOALS

ACTION STEPS	STATUS	✓
		☐
		☐
		☐
		☐

MILESTONES & REWARDS:

THOUGHTS & REFLECTIONS::

Weekly Priority List

MON	
TUE	
WED	
THUR	
FRI	
SAT	
SUN	

Checklist

FOR: _____   DATE: _____ ✓

_____   _____ ☐

_____   _____ ☐

_____   _____ ☐

_____   _____ ☐

_____   _____ ☐

_____   _____ ☐

_____   _____ ☐

_____   _____ ☐

_____   _____ ☐

_____   _____ ☐

_____   _____ ☐

_____   _____ ☐

_____   _____ ☐

_____   _____ ☐

_____   _____ ☐

NOTES:

Daily Planner

DATE

_____

TOP PRIORITIES:

MORNING:

AFTERNOON:

EVENING:

APPOINTMENTS:

NOTES:

GOALS FOR THE DAY::

Daily Planner

DATE
_____

TOP PRIORITIES:

MORNING:
....
_____
_____
_____

AFTERNOON:
....
_____
_____
....

APPOINTMENTS:

EVENING:
....
....
_____

NOTES:
....
....
....

GOALS FOR THE DAY::

Daily Planner

DATE

TOP PRIORITIES:

APPOINTMENTS:

GOALS FOR THE DAY::

MORNING:

AFTERNOON:

EVENING:

NOTES:

Daily Planner

DATE

TOP PRIORITIES:

APPOINTMENTS:

GOALS FOR THE DAY::

MORNING:

AFTERNOON:

EVENING:

NOTES:

Daily Planner

DATE

TOP PRIORITIES:

APPOINTMENTS:

GOALS FOR THE DAY::

MORNING:

AFTERNOON:

EVENING:

NOTES:

Daily Planner

DATE

TOP PRIORITIES:

APPOINTMENTS:

GOALS FOR THE DAY::

MORNING:

AFTERNOON:

EVENING:

NOTES:

Daily Planner

DATE

TOP PRIORITIES:

APPOINTMENTS:

GOALS FOR THE DAY::

MORNING:

AFTERNOON:

EVENING:

NOTES:

Weekly Snapshot

MON:

TUE:

WED:

THUR:

FRI:

SAT:

SUN:

TO DO LIST

NOTES

REMINDERS

My Action Plan

DATE:

TOP PRIORITIES

GOALS

ACTION STEPS

STATUS ✓

MILESTONES & REWARDS:

THOUGHTS & REFLECTIONS::

Weekly Priority List

MON	
TUE	
WED	
THUR	
FRI	
SAT	
SUN	

Checklist

FOR: _____   DATE: _____   ✓

_____   _____   ☐
_____   _____   ☐
_____   _____   ☐
_____   _____   ☐
_____   _____   ☐
_____   _____   ☐
_____   _____   ☐
_____   _____   ☐
_____   _____   ☐
_____   _____   ☐
_____   _____   ☐
_____   _____   ☐
_____   _____   ☐
_____   _____   ☐

NOTES:

Daily Planner

DATE

TOP PRIORITIES:

APPOINTMENTS:

GOALS FOR THE DAY::

MORNING:

AFTERNOON:

EVENING:

NOTES:

Daily Planner

DATE

_____

TOP PRIORITIES:

MORNING:

AFTERNOON:

APPOINTMENTS:

EVENING:

NOTES:

GOALS FOR THE DAY::

Daily Planner

DATE

TOP PRIORITIES:

APPOINTMENTS:

GOALS FOR THE DAY::

MORNING:

AFTERNOON:

EVENING:

NOTES:

Daily Planner

DATE

TOP PRIORITIES:

APPOINTMENTS:

GOALS FOR THE DAY::

MORNING:

AFTERNOON:

EVENING:

NOTES:

Daily Planner

DATE
_____

TOP PRIORITIES:

MORNING:
....
....
....

AFTERNOON:
....
....
....

APPOINTMENTS:

EVENING:
....
....
....

NOTES:
....
....
....

GOALS FOR THE DAY::

Daily Planner

DATE

TOP PRIORITIES:

APPOINTMENTS:

GOALS FOR THE DAY::

MORNING:

AFTERNOON:

EVENING:

NOTES:

Daily Planner

DATE

TOP PRIORITIES:

APPOINTMENTS:

GOALS FOR THE DAY::

MORNING:

AFTERNOON:

EVENING:

NOTES:

Weekly Snapshot

MON:

TUE:

WED:

THUR:

FRI:

SAT:

SUN:

TO DO LIST

NOTES

REMINDERS

My Action Plan

DATE:

TOP PRIORITIES

GOALS

ACTION STEPS	STATUS	✓
		☐
		☐
		☐
		☐

MILESTONES & REWARDS:

THOUGHTS & REFLECTIONS::

Weekly Priority List

MON	
TUE	
WED	
THUR	
FRI	
SAT	
SUN	

Checklist

FOR: DATE: ✓

NOTES:

Daily Planner

DATE

TOP PRIORITIES:

APPOINTMENTS:

GOALS FOR THE DAY::

MORNING:

AFTERNOON:

EVENING:

NOTES:

Daily Planner

DATE
_____

TOP PRIORITIES:

MORNING:
_____
_____
_____

AFTERNOON:
_____
_____
_____

APPOINTMENTS:

EVENING:
_____
_____
_____

NOTES:
_____
_____
_____

GOALS FOR THE DAY::

Daily Planner

DATE

TOP PRIORITIES:

APPOINTMENTS:

GOALS FOR THE DAY::

MORNING:

AFTERNOON:

EVENING:

NOTES:

Daily Planner

DATE

TOP PRIORITIES:

APPOINTMENTS:

GOALS FOR THE DAY::

MORNING:

AFTERNOON:

EVENING:

NOTES:

Daily Planner

DATE

TOP PRIORITIES:

APPOINTMENTS:

GOALS FOR THE DAY::

MORNING:

AFTERNOON:

EVENING:

NOTES:

Daily Planner

DATE

TOP PRIORITIES:

APPOINTMENTS:

GOALS FOR THE DAY::

MORNING:

AFTERNOON:

EVENING:

NOTES:

Daily Planner

DATE

TOP PRIORITIES:

APPOINTMENTS:

GOALS FOR THE DAY::

MORNING:

AFTERNOON:

EVENING:

NOTES:

Weekly Snapshot

MON:

TUE:

WED:

THUR:

FRI:

SAT:

SUN:

TO DO LIST

NOTES

REMINDERS

My Action Plan

DATE:

TOP PRIORITIES	GOALS

ACTION STEPS	STATUS	✓
		▢
		▢
		▢
		▢

MILESTONES & REWARDS:

THOUGHTS & REFLECTIONS::

Weekly Priority List

MON	
TUE	
WED	
THUR	
FRI	
SAT	
SUN	

Checklist

FOR: | DATE: | ✓

NOTES:

Daily Planner

DATE

TOP PRIORITIES:

APPOINTMENTS:

GOALS FOR THE DAY::

MORNING:

AFTERNOON:

EVENING:

NOTES:

Daily Planner

DATE

MORNING:

TOP PRIORITIES:

AFTERNOON:

APPOINTMENTS:

EVENING:

NOTES:

GOALS FOR THE DAY::

Daily Planner

DATE
_____

TOP PRIORITIES:

MORNING:

AFTERNOON:

EVENING:

APPOINTMENTS:

NOTES:

GOALS FOR THE DAY::

Daily Planner

DATE

TOP PRIORITIES:

APPOINTMENTS:

GOALS FOR THE DAY::

MORNING:

AFTERNOON:

EVENING:

NOTES:

Daily Planner

DATE

TOP PRIORITIES:

APPOINTMENTS:

GOALS FOR THE DAY::

MORNING:

AFTERNOON:

EVENING:

NOTES:

Daily Planner

DATE

TOP PRIORITIES:

APPOINTMENTS:

GOALS FOR THE DAY::

MORNING:

AFTERNOON:

EVENING:

NOTES:

Daily Planner

DATE

TOP PRIORITIES:

APPOINTMENTS:

GOALS FOR THE DAY::

MORNING:

AFTERNOON:

EVENING:

NOTES:

Weekly Snapshot

MON:

TUE:

WED:

THUR:

FRI:

SAT:

SUN:

TO DO LIST

NOTES

REMINDERS

My Action Plan

DATE:

TOP PRIORITIES	GOALS

ACTION STEPS   STATUS   ✓

MILESTONES & REWARDS:

THOUGHTS & REFLECTIONS::

Weekly Priority List

MON	
TUE	
WED	
THUR	
FRI	
SAT	
SUN	

Checklist

FOR: _____   DATE: _____   ✓

_____ _____ ☐
_____ _____ ☐
_____ _____ ☐
_____ _____ ☐
_____ _____ ☐
_____ _____ ☐
_____ _____ ☐
_____ _____ ☐
_____ _____ ☐
_____ _____ ☐
_____ _____ ☐
_____ _____ ☐
_____ _____ ☐
_____ _____ ☐

NOTES:

Daily Planner

DATE

TOP PRIORITIES:

APPOINTMENTS:

GOALS FOR THE DAY::

MORNING:

AFTERNOON:

EVENING:

NOTES:

Daily Planner

DATE

TOP PRIORITIES:

APPOINTMENTS:

GOALS FOR THE DAY::

MORNING:

AFTERNOON:

EVENING:

NOTES:

Daily Planner

DATE

_____

TOP PRIORITIES:

MORNING:

AFTERNOON:

EVENING:

APPOINTMENTS:

NOTES:

GOALS FOR THE DAY::

Daily Planner

DATE

TOP PRIORITIES:

APPOINTMENTS:

GOALS FOR THE DAY::

MORNING:

AFTERNOON:

EVENING:

NOTES:

Daily Planner

DATE

TOP PRIORITIES:

APPOINTMENTS:

GOALS FOR THE DAY::

MORNING:

AFTERNOON:

EVENING:

NOTES:

Daily Planner

DATE

TOP PRIORITIES:

APPOINTMENTS:

GOALS FOR THE DAY::

MORNING:

AFTERNOON:

EVENING:

NOTES:

Daily Planner

DATE

TOP PRIORITIES:

APPOINTMENTS:

GOALS FOR THE DAY::

MORNING:

AFTERNOON:

EVENING:

NOTES:

Weekly Snapshot

MON:

TUE:

WED:

THUR:

FRI:

SAT:

SUN:

TO DO LIST

NOTES

REMINDERS

My Action Plan

DATE:

TOP PRIORITIES

GOALS

ACTION STEPS

STATUS ✓

MILESTONES & REWARDS:

THOUGHTS & REFLECTIONS::

Weekly Priority List

MON	
TUE	
WED	
THUR	
FRI	
SAT	
SUN	

Checklist

FOR: DATE: ✓

_____   _____

_____   _____

_____   _____

_____   _____

_____   _____

_____   _____

_____   _____

_____   _____

_____   _____

_____   _____

_____   _____

_____   _____

_____   _____

_____   _____

NOTES:

Daily Planner

DATE

TOP PRIORITIES:

APPOINTMENTS:

GOALS FOR THE DAY::

MORNING:

AFTERNOON:

EVENING:

NOTES:

Daily Planner

DATE
_____

TOP PRIORITIES:

MORNING:
_____
_____
_____

AFTERNOON:
_____
_____
_____

APPOINTMENTS:

EVENING:
_____
_____
_____

NOTES:
_____
_____
_____

GOALS FOR THE DAY::

Daily Planner

DATE

MORNING:

TOP PRIORITIES:

AFTERNOON:

EVENING:

APPOINTMENTS:

NOTES:

GOALS FOR THE DAY::

Daily Planner

DATE

MORNING:

TOP PRIORITIES:

AFTERNOON:

APPOINTMENTS:

EVENING:

NOTES:

GOALS FOR THE DAY::

Daily Planner

DATE

MORNING:

TOP PRIORITIES:

AFTERNOON:

EVENING:

APPOINTMENTS:

NOTES:

GOALS FOR THE DAY::

Daily Planner

DATE
_____

TOP PRIORITIES:

APPOINTMENTS:

GOALS FOR THE DAY::

MORNING:

AFTERNOON:

EVENING:

NOTES:

Daily Planner

DATE

TOP PRIORITIES:

APPOINTMENTS:

MORNING:

AFTERNOON:

EVENING:

NOTES:

GOALS FOR THE DAY::

Weekly Snapshot

MON:

TUE:

WED:

THUR:

FRI:

SAT:

SUN:

TO DO LIST

NOTES

REMINDERS

My Action Plan

DATE:

TOP PRIORITIES	GOALS

ACTION STEPS   STATUS   ✓

_____   _____   ☐

_____   _____   ☐

_____   _____   ☐

_____   _____   ☐

MILESTONES & REWARDS:

THOUGHTS & REFLECTIONS::

Weekly Priority List

MON	
TUE	
WED	
THUR	
FRI	
SAT	
SUN	

Checklist

FOR: _____   DATE: _____   ✓

NOTES:

Daily Planner

DATE

TOP PRIORITIES:

APPOINTMENTS:

GOALS FOR THE DAY::

MORNING:

AFTERNOON:

EVENING:

NOTES:

Daily Planner

DATE

TOP PRIORITIES:

APPOINTMENTS:

MORNING:

AFTERNOON:

EVENING:

NOTES:

GOALS FOR THE DAY::

Daily Planner

DATE

TOP PRIORITIES:

APPOINTMENTS:

GOALS FOR THE DAY::

MORNING:

AFTERNOON:

EVENING:

NOTES:

Daily Planner

DATE

TOP PRIORITIES:

APPOINTMENTS:

MORNING:

AFTERNOON:

EVENING:

NOTES:

GOALS FOR THE DAY::

Daily Planner

DATE

_____

TOP PRIORITIES:

APPOINTMENTS:

GOALS FOR THE DAY::

MORNING:

AFTERNOON:

EVENING:

NOTES:

Daily Planner

DATE

TOP PRIORITIES:

APPOINTMENTS:

GOALS FOR THE DAY::

MORNING:

AFTERNOON:

EVENING:

NOTES:

Daily Planner

DATE

TOP PRIORITIES:

APPOINTMENTS:

GOALS FOR THE DAY::

MORNING:

AFTERNOON:

EVENING:

NOTES:

Weekly Snapshot

MON:

TUE:

WED:

THUR:

FRI:

SAT:

SUN:

TO DO LIST

NOTES

REMINDERS

My Action Plan

DATE:

TOP PRIORITIES

GOALS

ACTION STEPS	STATUS	✓

MILESTONES & REWARDS:

THOUGHTS & REFLECTIONS::

Weekly Priority List

MON	
TUE	
WED	
THUR	
FRI	
SAT	
SUN	

Checklist

FOR:

DATE:

✓

NOTES:

Daily Planner

DATE

TOP PRIORITIES:

APPOINTMENTS:

GOALS FOR THE DAY::

MORNING:

AFTERNOON:

EVENING:

NOTES:

Daily Planner

DATE

TOP PRIORITIES:

APPOINTMENTS:

GOALS FOR THE DAY::

MORNING:

AFTERNOON:

EVENING:

NOTES:

Daily Planner

DATE

MORNING:

TOP PRIORITIES:

AFTERNOON:

APPOINTMENTS:

EVENING:

NOTES:

GOALS FOR THE DAY::

Daily Planner

DATE

TOP PRIORITIES:

APPOINTMENTS:

GOALS FOR THE DAY::

MORNING:

AFTERNOON:

EVENING:

NOTES:

Daily Planner

DATE

_____

TOP PRIORITIES:

MORNING:
_____
_____
_____
_____

AFTERNOON:
_____
_____
_____

APPOINTMENTS:

EVENING:
_____
_____

NOTES:
_____
_____
_____

GOALS FOR THE DAY::

Daily Planner

DATE

TOP PRIORITIES:

APPOINTMENTS:

GOALS FOR THE DAY::

MORNING:

AFTERNOON:

EVENING:

NOTES:

Daily Planner

DATE

TOP PRIORITIES:

APPOINTMENTS:

MORNING:

AFTERNOON:

EVENING:

NOTES:

GOALS FOR THE DAY::

Weekly Snapshot

MON:

TUE:

WED:

THUR:

FRI:

SAT:

SUN:

TO DO LIST

NOTES

REMINDERS

My Action Plan

DATE:

TOP PRIORITIES	GOALS

ACTION STEPS	STATUS	✓
		▪
		▪
		▪
		▪

MILESTONES & REWARDS:

THOUGHTS & REFLECTIONS::

Weekly Priority List

MON	
TUE	
WED	
THUR	
FRI	
SAT	
SUN	

Checklist

FOR: _____   DATE: _____   ✓

_____   _____   ▢

_____   _____   ▢

_____   _____   ▢

_____   _____   ▢

_____   _____   ▢

_____   _____   ▢

_____   _____   ▢

_____   _____   ▢

_____   _____   ▢

_____   _____   ▢

_____   _____   ▢

_____   _____   ▢

_____   _____   ▢

_____   _____   ▢

_____   _____   ▢

NOTES:

Daily Planner

DATE

TOP PRIORITIES:

APPOINTMENTS:

GOALS FOR THE DAY::

MORNING:

AFTERNOON:

EVENING:

NOTES:

Daily Planner

DATE

_____

TOP PRIORITIES:

MORNING:

AFTERNOON:

EVENING:

APPOINTMENTS:

NOTES:

GOALS FOR THE DAY::

Daily Planner

DATE

TOP PRIORITIES:

APPOINTMENTS:

GOALS FOR THE DAY::

MORNING:

AFTERNOON:

EVENING:

NOTES:

Daily Planner

DATE
_____

TOP PRIORITIES:

MORNING:
_____
_____
_____

AFTERNOON:
_____
_____
_____

APPOINTMENTS:

EVENING:
_____
_____

NOTES:
_____
_____
_____

GOALS FOR THE DAY::

Daily Planner

DATE

TOP PRIORITIES:

APPOINTMENTS:

GOALS FOR THE DAY::

MORNING:

AFTERNOON:

EVENING:

NOTES:

Daily Planner

DATE

TOP PRIORITIES:

APPOINTMENTS:

GOALS FOR THE DAY::

MORNING:

AFTERNOON:

EVENING:

NOTES:

Daily Planner

DATE

TOP PRIORITIES:

APPOINTMENTS:

GOALS FOR THE DAY::

MORNING:

AFTERNOON:

EVENING:

NOTES:

Daily Planner

DATE

TOP PRIORITIES:

APPOINTMENTS:

GOALS FOR THE DAY::

MORNING:

AFTERNOON:

EVENING:

NOTES:

Daily Planner

DATE

TOP PRIORITIES:

APPOINTMENTS:

GOALS FOR THE DAY::

MORNING:

AFTERNOON:

EVENING:

NOTES:

Made in the USA
Coppell, TX
13 June 2024

33479007R00070